Why We Haven't Cured Cancer:

How Biomedical Research ~~Works~~ In America Today

Dr. Carl S. Bucky

Why We Haven't Cured Cancer

All rights reserved

Copyright Carl S. Bucky

Bethesda, MD

December, 2011

ISBN-13: 978-1469901886

ISBN-10: 1469901889

Dedication

This book is for the researchers who have dedicated their lives to fighting cancer. I wish a system existed that would support you in your work.

Introduction   5

Section 1: The Realms of Research

1. Academic Labs   11
2. Big Pharma   34
3. Government Labs   45

Section 2: Where Does the Money Go?

4. Scientific Equipment and Supplies   68
5. Publishing   78
6. The Work Force   92

7. Why We Haven't Cured Cancer   96

Why We Haven't Cured Cancer

Introduction

I always wanted to be a scientist. Actually, I'll rephrase that statement. From the time that I accepted that I would never be a grizzly bear, I always wanted to be a scientist. When I got those thick-rimmed glasses in 3rd grade, I even looked the part. At first, my goal was to be an archaeologist. What other scientist does a kid in a rural village in the mountains even know about? My focus changed in 5th grade, however, when my aunt went to her doctor complaining of stomach pains and died of colon cancer 6 short days later. Incidentally, she was the same age as I am now as I sit here typing this.

The day after her funeral I decided that I would cure cancer. I spent every waking moment that summer trying to find out everything I could about the disease from the old Encyclopedia Britannica I had won in the state spelling bee that year. This opened up to me the idea that scientists can do more than explore the past – they can open the door to the future with new treatments and cures. A couple of decades later, I sit here typing in my apartment sick with the knowledge that after all the years of work on this disease we are really no closer to curing cancer than we were when I was 10 years old.

Why We Haven't Cured Cancer

Why haven't we gotten there yet? Why is there still a threat that could randomly strike any person you or I love at almost any second and take them from our lives? Why is our life expectancy actually shorter now after the diagnosis of some cancers than it was 70 years ago? Why hasn't there been a major breakthrough in my lifetime? Why are we still using the same treatments that were in use when my grandfather was my age?

One answer is that cancer is simply one of the most complex diseases in existence. It can arise from a short-circuiting of any number of processes occurring within our own cells, when mechanisms that normally protect us fail in the worst possible way. While this is undoubtedly the truth, there is another less obvious answer. The system of biomedical research in America today is so poorly designed that the only possible outcome is failure.

Every year billions of dollars are allocated for cancer research. One government agency heavily involved in this research has a budget of about $5 billion dollars per year. This is only one agency and doesn't include the millions of dollars produced by independent entities and non-profit organizations that are set aside for improving treatment for cancer, or even the budgets set aside for research in other developed nations. And what do we have to show for decades of work and this mind boggling amount of money? A 2% decrease in annual mortality rates from cancer over the last 40 years. Even this number is questionable. Is the 2% decrease due to advances in cancer treatment or the fact that over this same time period the percentage of cigarette smokers in the U.S. has dropped from 40% to around 20% (as of 2007 CDC numbers)? I believe the decrease in smoking and the increase in atherosclerosis as a cause of death in the U.S. contribute more to the decrease in cancer deaths than any improvement in cancer treatment that has occurred over the past 40 years.

There is a simple formula in research that has been shown to produce results. This formula has worked in every major scientific development in history and requires that three criteria are met. The first is that you need a workforce of the most highly skilled individuals working on the task. Ideally, these workers must be young enough to bring new ideas to the table, but old enough to have learned what approaches have failed in the past. The second is that the workers must have incentive to succeed in this task. The third requirement is that these workers must have the resources necessary to succeed in their task.

One great example of this is the race to the moon. Over the 20 year push to beat the Russians into space we were able to meet all three criteria. We had an entire generation of the best scientists and engineers on earth working together. Due to the enthusiasm for this project and the income, job stability, and prominence associated with being an engineer for the space program, we were able to choose the best and the brightest for the task. The amount of money allotted for the program was sufficient to launch many rockets and incremental improvements in technology and protocols allowed us to finally place the feet of twelve astronauts on the moon. Other examples exist as well, including the Manhattan project and the amazing number of vaccines created in the mid-20th century that eradicated such terrible scourges to humanity as polio and yellow fever.

The system responsible for cancer research, however, does not meet any of these criteria. How can that be when we allot billions of dollars to eradicating this disease? As I'll detail in the following chapters the money we think is going toward cancer research and innovative cancer researchers is not reaching the intended targets. Instead, it is being misallocated by politically motivated individuals and being swallowed up by greedy universities and corporations. Curing cancer is often only an afterthought in the use of these funds.

I have chosen to publish this work anonymously in order to protect my career, my family and my coworkers from the ramifications of the truths I will reveal about the system I have worked in for the majority of my life. Although details in this book have been changed in order to maintain my anonymity, all of the facts and stories revealed in these pages are true.

Section 1: The Three Realms of Research

Before we go further, it is important to separate the three realms of biomedical research. The role of scientists and the fate of the money allocated for cancer research are divided between these three groups. Academic research labs are operated by professors at colleges and universities, primarily using student and trainee labor. The research at academic labs is funded by federal and private grants. Private pharmaceutical companies, or Big Pharma, are for-profit entities that study cancer with the goal of producing treatments and chemotherapy agents that they can sell to support further research and keep their stockholders smiling. The final realm, government, performs research using taxpayer money, often in large central facilities in or near major cities. The goal of these massive facilities is the eradication of cancer for the benefit of the U.S. population.

Chapter 1: Academic labs

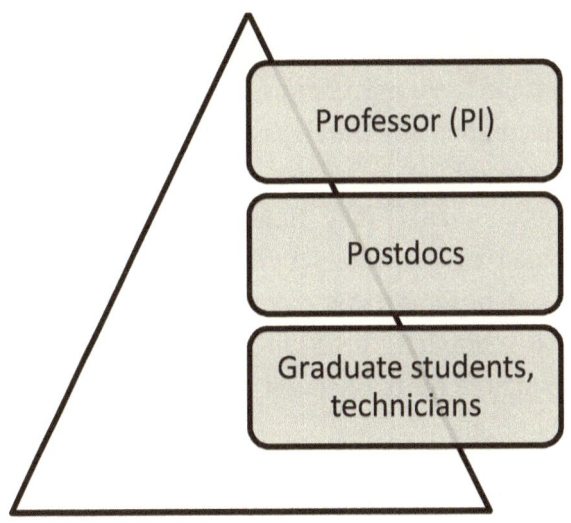

The figure above is a schematic describing your typical academic lab. In this setup, the Professor (also called a Principal Investigator, or PI) is the ruler. In an ideal situation, the PI is a mentor to the people under him/her, can obtain grant money to keep the lab functioning, and provides support and guidance to his/her students and postdoctoral fellows.

At the bottom of the food chain are the graduate students. These are the cheapest labor. In order to be accepted into graduate school, these students must obtain bachelor's degrees in Biology, Chemistry, or related sciences. Most schools will not accept graduate students who earned grade-point-averages below 3.5 on a 4 point scale. Most graduate students work as graduate teaching assistants (GTAs), teaching undergraduate courses at the large universities. A few fortunate ones work as graduate research assistants (GRAs) and perform research to earn their salaries. On top of these assignments, they must complete a hefty course load of graduate level science courses, form and suitably impress a committee of professors, as well as complete between 1 to 3 research projects suitable for publication in a peer-reviewed scientific journal.

Students completing their Master's degrees typically complete one project. Students working on their doctorates at most institutions also have to complete a Preliminary Examination in their 2nd or 3rd year. These exams vary between institutions. Some schools require both lengthy written and oral examinations. Despite the format, the outcome is typically the same. Students who pass this examination are allowed to continue to work toward their Doctorates, students who fail are allowed to complete a Master's degree, or asked to leave the institution at the end of the current term.

A few years ago, the idea began circulating that Master's students do not produce as much, on average, as Doctoral students during their studies. The idea goes: it takes 1-2 years to train a graduate student to do research. By the time the Master's students are trained, they only produce around 1 year of useful research. Doctoral students, however, provide useful research for 3-5 years. As a consequence, most large universities no longer recruit Master's students. In order to get a Master's degree in one of the biomedical sciences, it is often necessary to apply to a Doctoral program, and either fail your preliminary examination or get special permission from your advisory committee after you have put a few years of work into your research.

For doctoral students who successfully complete their preliminary examination, the work is hardly over. Although they have typically completed their course work by this time, they still have teaching and research responsibilities, as well as working to complete a dissertation and those 1 to 3 publications. During my graduate work, I think I worked an average of about 70 hours a week. This is more than some, and less than others, but I think my experience is fairly typical. For my work I earned $14,000 plus my tuition my first year, 2004 (although I still had to pay $2,000 in student fees). After obtaining every possible merit-based pay increase available at the University, my final year I made $16,500 (but student fees had been increased to roughly $3,000). Although the rates for graduate stipends have increased over the years, to this day the highest stipend I've ever heard of was $26,000, and that was for a university in Washington, D.C.

Fortunately for me and other graduate students, the Department of Education is very liberal in providing student loans for post-graduate studies. Unfortunately, this leads to many people being completely submerged in student loan debt by the time they complete their degrees. According to the National Post-Secondary Student Aid Study (NPSAS) the average graduate of a Ph.D. program accrues around $70,000 in student loan debt. Compare this to the $20,000 borrowed by the average graduate of a bachelor's program (data as of 2008).

If you are fortunate, and chose a good advisor and research committee, the academic system can work well for you. You learn far more about your subject area than you possibly could have in any other way. You publish some original experiments, learning over the years all the secrets of the craft and get to network with other scientists in order to begin shaping your plans for the future. You learn about the various realms of research, the benefits and problems with each, and get a general idea of your career goals and how to achieve them.

If you are really unfortunate, you spend years toiling under an oppressive advisor and research committee. You fund your own research through small grants and by teaching a full course load. Around these responsibilities you don't receive good guidance on your research projects and you never publish anything (or anything valuable). Since you have to raise your own money you never attend conferences and don't get to network with other scientists, meaning that you graduate unknown to the scientific community and without any proof that you can actually perform a scientific study.

While most students' experiences fall between these two extremes, a surprising degree of your early professional success depends on how fortunate you are. If you interviewed with 3 professors at different universities, and you pick the wrong one, you may be handicapped for the rest of your career. Even knowing that, I know that I'd prefer to hire someone who finished their Ph.D. in 4 years and published 3 papers over someone who spent 7 years on their degree and completed only 1 paper. While first student *may* have worked much harder than the second student, it is almost impossible to know the situation faced by each one. The first student may have been on a research fellowship, as I was, throughout their entire degree. As such they would have more time to research and always have funding to perform experiments. The second student may have had to teach all 14 semesters. Unfortunately, there currently is no way to distinguish between these two students, except that the first one is much more likely to land a nice postdoctoral fellowship.

While in graduate school, a fellow student on the edge of my circle of acquaintances fell into an even worse scenario than my worst-case described above. In his fourth year, while preparing his first publication, his advisor was fired. I don't know what he did, but the rumors all suggested that it was pretty bad, and he was terminated immediately. This left his student in a nightmare scenario. With too much invested to quit, or even to accept a Master's degree, he was forced to join any lab that would take him. While he was able to complete his primary study on animal viruses, he had to spend an additional three years working in a plant disease lab; this was the only lab on campus with the funding to take a student in the middle of a semester.

As I mention later in this book, I recently switched careers. Even though I was leaving the seventh lab of my career for my eighth, the hiring committee required a letter of recommendation from my graduate advisor. This is a common requirement of academic research jobs. Not only is it important that you perform good research, good teaching, and publish original scientific data, it is crucial that your advisor likes and respects you enough to write letters of recommendation for you throughout your career. If your advisor does not, consider yourself sunk.

It is impossible to imagine that this power isn't abused from time to time. Your research advisor has the power to decide whether you get a degree, whether you get paid (and commonly, how much or little) during that degree, and on top of that has the power to weigh in on your promotion to that new lab. With the cards stacked in this way, I hope that every student who goes into higher education in the sciences is as fortunate as I was, though I have certainly heard enough anecdotes to know that not everyone is so lucky.

Postdoctoral Fellows

During the final year of a Ph.D., you are often required to obtain a suitable postdoctoral appointment in order to finally graduate. It is virtually impossible to land any position other than a postdoc directly after graduate school. Unfortunately, once you start your postdoctoral appointment you have to start paying back your student loans. With a Ph.D., surely your salary is high enough to take care of pesky student loans, right? In 2011 a lab I was working in hired a postdoc who told us that his next highest salary offer was $27,000 per year. Later, he admitted to me that he wanted that job more than the one he accepted with us but he couldn't figure out how to buy diapers for his newborn on that salary. The NIH sets guidelines each year for postdoctoral salaries for labs that currently have grant support from the federal government. For 1st year postdocs, the salary is supposed to be around $36,000. Realistically, the NIH does not enforce this rule; it is simply a guideline they would like you to follow. Strangely enough, if you work inside the NIH itself, the starting pay for postdocs is currently around $45,000.

An important aspect of the postdoctoral fellowship is the complete absence of any form of basic labor laws. Postdocs are completely at the mercy of their PI when it comes to vacation time, sick leave, and hours worked per week. In the most respected universities, postdocs typically work in excess of 70 hours per week to meet the expectations of their advisors. During my first postdoc, my advisor expected me to be at work at 7 a.m. Monday-Friday and my wife commonly beat me home when she got off work at 11 p.m. I didn't have an entire weekend off in order to make the trip to visit my family, except for the holidays, during my entire fellowship. And don't think I was the only one.

Other postdocs on my floor beat me to work and were still at their bench when I left.

Ask any researcher about their postdoc experience and you will hear nightmares of PIs who abused their power and their employees. One of my favorite stories is from one of my professors in graduate school. During his postdoc at one of the Universities of California in the 1980s, his advisor would fire all of his postdocs for one day each year before hiring them back the next day. Due to this procedure, he didn't have to provide his postdocs with the state-mandated health insurance plan, nor did he have to justify why they never received pay raises. In another example, a prominent professor at a very famous college is infamous for never giving his postdocs good letters of recommendation, effectively trapping them in his laboratory. The better the postdoc, the less likely he will ever let them leave. Eventually his advisees either accept permanent, low-paying Associate positions in his lab, or they drop out of science completely.

Again, these are only anecdotes and I hope these do not represent the experiences of the majority of researchers. But it is important to note that these situations can and do occur and may be inevitable in a system that gives one person such encompassing power over the fate of another.

In the system I have described, where does the ingenuity come from to develop new technology, new techniques, and new ideas? Does it come from the graduate student who is taking classes, teaching classes and squeezing in research around dodging bill collectors because he or she cannot pay their car insurance on their $14,000 stipend?

Perhaps the new, great ideas come from the postdocs? Nothing fosters ingenuity and creativity like sleep deprivation and working under high stress conditions. Around the 6 to 7 day work-week, the frequent late notices on the $800 student loan payments, rent and child care for the poor child who never sees its parent, there doesn't seem to be a lot of time for ingenuity to me.

Of course, the ideas must come from the professors, who have finally made it to the promise land of 8 hours of sleep each night and financial security!

Professors

By method of elimination, we have identified the ideal professors. These amazing people were able to avoid partying in college and graduate at the head of their class in a difficult field of science. Instead of taking a secure job, they opted to apply to a prestigious graduate program. Once surrounded by their peers, they managed to survive their preliminary exams, teach and do research for 4 to 6 years and earned their Ph.D. Following their Ph.D. they accepted a Postdoctoral Fellowship in an even more prestigious lab and in 2-5 years successfully wrote grants and amazing papers that made it into the very best academic journals. After all this work, they were able to convince a major university to make an investment in their dreams and research program. The good times are surely ahead.

A few years ago I served on a selection committee for a new professor in my field of study for a major university. The competition was fierce. We interviewed applicants from Harvard, Princeton, U.C. Berkley, and other prominent schools. Each applicant spent 2 full days on campus delivering seminars and eventually shook the hand of nearly every person on the entire campus. Next, we gathered the opinions of every person who heard Dr. So-and-so speak or met with him/her. Next came the crucial part, we looked at their academic publications and the impact factors of the journals they published in. An impact factor is a mostly arbitrary system of ranking the prominence associated with publishing a paper in a specific academic research journal. There are around 10 systems for ranking journals, and every field of study has their favorite one. If you do an internet search for 'name of journal' and 'impact factor' you will find that each journal has its favorite system as well, typically the one that gives them their journal the biggest number.

Taking these numbers, we used the following system: If you were listed as the first or last author on a paper, then we gave you the impact factor of that journal. In other words, if your name was the first one in order of the listed authors and your paper was published in a journal with an impact factor of 10, then you got 10 points. Same if you were the last author. First author status commonly indicates that all the authors agreed that you had the most to do with this paper. Last author status generally means that this work occurred in your lab or under your guidance. There are exceptions to these rules, but this is basically the system we used.

If you were 2nd, 3rd, 4th, or 17th author and there were no special notes saying that you 'contributed equally' to the paper along with the first author, we used a different equation. We counted up the number of authors and divided the impact factor of the journal by the number of authors. For example, if you were the 2nd author out of 10 total authors and you published this paper in a journal with an impact factor of 10, then we divided 10 by 10 and gave you 1 impact factor point for this publication. I've mentioned this system in passing to other researchers at other institutions and this system doesn't seem out of the ordinary at all. My guess is that most big universities do something similar to gauge the prominence of their applicants. I'll call this the prominence quotient, or PQ.

Again, the PQ was just one criterion we used during the selection process. The amount of grant money you had successfully brought in by this point in your career was another big one. The third big criterion was the basis of your research: are you studying something interesting that will bring in big dollars? Each year, government granting agencies outline key objectives that they would like to focus on. If you work in one of these high impact areas there is often more grant money available for you to perform your research. For example, following the anthrax attacks of 2001, researchers with experience working with anthrax had more opportunities to secure research funding, as all of the funding agencies placed bioterrorism as key objectives.

At the end of all this investigation, we had ranked our applicants in order of who would be the most prominent addition to the faculty and would have the greatest chance of bringing money into the school. We brought this list of recommendations to the university's governing body. After carefully reviewing our recommendations and the results of our weeks of work, one clever member of the governing board noticed this fact: only one of the seven applicants was female. Decision made.

I'm going to step back for a second here. I am not against equality in the workforce at all. We need protections in place to protect us from discrimination, both the blatant kind and the subconscious kind that we often don't know we're doing. I know that as hard as it was for me to get through to where I am in life, it would have been significantly harder if I had to do it without being a tall white Caucasian. Take away any of those 3 descriptors and I may not be sitting where I am now. This is my complaint: As a committee, which had an equal male to female ratio, we developed a system that attempted to determine, impartially, who was the best candidate for the position at their university, when all along we should have said 'only 1 woman applied, obviously it is her job.' The gap between the top candidate and the applicant who was hired was rather large; in fact, she was the one we ranked 7th out of 7. I still have acquaintances at that university, and by all accounts the new professor is doing quite well. However, I still believe that our selection could have been made in a more scientific manner and increased the chances of our selection succeeding, but we will never know.

Tenure

So you're now an Assistant Professor! You now have the easy job. You're job requirements are only to teach undergraduate and graduate level courses, mentor undergraduates (usually the number of students in your program divided by the number of professors, so somewhere between 20 and 200), construct a laboratory capable of attracting extramural funding, write papers, write grants, and perform service for your university. By service, they mean extra things to support the university and your department. A normal job description for a professor will say something like 40:50:10, as the ratio between teaching, research and service. In other words you have 2 full-time jobs as a professor/mentor and the manager of a research facility. Around these responsibilities you should also organize barbeques for the faculty, provide supervision to a couple of university organizations, and maybe host a conference where people can come to see the work of your department's graduate students. Hopefully you don't have a family that would like to see you.

On the up-side, at least now you have a respectable salary. The professor we 'chose' for the position I described above had the amazing income of $58,000 per year. This isn't ancient history, either. This hire was made in 2008. And this wasn't a small college; this was one of the largest universities in the U.S.

Okay, so you're still working 80+ hours/ week, and still worrying about those 10+ years of student loans. So what? At least you have job security. Oh wait. You'll have job security, when you are granted tenure. Tenure is awarded to assistant professors when they have proven themselves to be assets to their university. This generally means that you've brought in substantial sums of grant money, as well as published some impressive papers out of your new lab, as well as provided invaluable services to your department. Who determines when you've earned tenure? Obviously, the professors who have already earned it do. In the past, most colleges allowed you 6-7 years to earn tenure. If you haven't received tenure by that deadline, you are simply released by the university.

A recent trend at the 'best' research institutions is to shorten the deadline for tenure to 3 years. This is particularly common when a job description is something like 10:80:10 for the ratio of teaching to research to service. In this situation you have only time to write grants and try to boost your profile in order to get grants. Accepting a position in a 3 year tenure situation is a big gamble. If you don't make tenure, you're dreams of being an academic professor are certainly over. Nothing will send your resume to the trash can as rapidly as having to list that you were denied tenure by another institution.

Grants

As mentioned above, in order to survive in academia, you need to bring in grant money. This money may come from one of the major government institutions, such as the NIH, USDA, or DOD. If you are studying a specific disease, you may also be able to obtain funding from private funds or from non-profit organizations. Grant applications are typically written requesting money for anywhere between a few thousand and a few million dollars. They may provide funding for anywhere from 1 to 7 years for your research program. What do you need in order to write an effective grant? First of all, you need preliminary data suggesting that your experiments will yield the results that you intend. For example, if you are studying a new chemotherapy agent that you invented and you want to see if it works on mice with cancer, you need two things. 1) To have invented the agent. 2) To have shown that it worked on mice with cancer.

Let's think about this. Essentially, you are writing a grant to get funding for something you've already done. Imagine you are a new assistant professor and you have 3-7 years to obtain grant funding. The first thing you want to do is start writing grants to fund your research, correct? No. The first thing you want to do is to rapidly set up your lab, hire graduate students and postdocs, train them and get to work on projects that may or may not attract funding. Sounds a little like gambling, doesn't it? You need to find a project that is interesting, feasible, and finish it so you get funding. If you fail at this point, as many do (especially in 3 year tenure environments), you and everyone you hired are going to be out of work very soon.

In order to get a grant you must apply to a government or public agency for the money. The grant application process is extremely thorough and since thousands of labs often apply for grants that can be issued to, at most, a few dozen researchers, the competition is fierce. In order to filter through all of these applications, a grant committee is established. These committees are made of the very best field leaders who don't mind giving up their weekends to read other people's research. Primarily these are young researchers who are trying to get their name circulated, and in my experience, they are almost completely made up of researchers who are unmarried. Every grant committee that I have ever heard of has the same first-level filtering technique, the typo filter. Regardless of the merit of the study, when there are hundreds of applications to look through, elimination of the 60% that have typographical or obvious grammatical errors definitely speeds up the process. The remaining applications are painstakingly studied and voted on by the committee. This is where making enemies during your career catches up to you.

Who gets grants? One kind of NIH grant is called an R01 grant. These are the very best kind as they supply uninterrupted funding for 4-7 years. A few years ago, someone sat down and did this calculation: the average scientist makes the most important discovery of their career in their early- to mid-thirties and the average scientist receives their first R01 grant in their early- to mid- forties. This is due to the amount of data that is necessary to write the large and imposing application for an R01. It takes years to come up with enough preliminary data to sell one of these grants. This has led to a very strange habit among field-leading researchers: the writing of grant applications for work that has already been fully completed. I know of several big-name guys who do this. You use your last grant to complete a research study and then you put it in your desk drawer. When the next grant application comes out, you use the completed study in your drawer to write the grant. It is easy to sell the study as feasible because you already successfully pulled it off! Once you get the grant you submit the paper and the grant committee is very impressed by how efficient you are. You use the remainder of the grant money to complete whatever project you feel like and when it is finished you write the next grant application.

This is obviously not the system that was intended, but due to a complete lack of regulation, this is the system we now have in place. This system rewards researchers who are essentially past the primes of their careers and provides the most funding to the researchers who bend the rules of the grant system.

Once you have received your grant, the funds are sent to your college or University, which takes a percentage to pay the bills, with these funds going toward electricity, water, toilet paper, and other things your lab uses that you don't think about. Typically the percentage the university takes for these incidental costs are about 50% - 70% of the total. You write a grant for your project which you expect to cost $1 million over the next three years. Your lab actually receives $300,000 of that million. So, if you need $1 million for your project, you actually write the grant for $2 - $3 million dollars. In case you were wondering, yes, scientists only use toilet paper made out of solid gold.

A few years ago a letter was written to the editors of *Science* magazine from an irate professor who discovered that a large portion of his grant was being used to support his University's art department. The editor responded that not only was this use of these funds legal, but the practice is becoming increasingly common. Universities have complete control over the use of funds that they declare as incidental expenses on grants received by researchers at their facilities. Whether it's a $10,000 grant from a non-profit organization or a $10 million dollar R01 award from the NIH that was meant to support the work of 10 postdocs developing chemotherapeutics for pancreatic cancer, the majority of this money may actually be going to purchase art supplies.

Who Gets To the Top?

Let's look at this system again. We start with high school students who have an interest in the biomedical sciences. In general, biology is a reasonably easy major to get in to. Biological science departments aren't typically as selective as engineering programs, for example. As a result, you are starting with a relatively large pool of biology graduates. Since most graduate schools require a 3.0 or 3.5 on a 4.0 scale for admissions, only the top one-third of biology degree recipients are eligible to begin graduate school, which narrows the pool a bit. A second requirement is that you must be willing to spend more time in school, when jobs as technicians are both available, and pay much more than graduate school. I'm sure that this has more to do with narrowing down the pool than the grade requirements.

Once in graduate school, you have many opportunities to fail. With graduate level science courses, a strict GPA limit, and preliminary exams, any mistake you make could seriously jeopardize your career in academia. If you make it through these pitfalls, you must still perform high quality original research for publications, as well as your thesis. Not meeting these requirements ends your chances of obtaining your Ph.D.

After getting this degree you have to put up with even more, low paying work, often without basic benefits such as vacation time and sick leave. If you aren't distracted by the higher pay available in the private and government sectors AND you publish some groundbreaking research AND you belong to the correct demographic a University is looking for - you have finally made it. And you get to keep your job if you are willing to subject yourself to more hours of volunteer service, teaching, and research while obtaining grant money from biomedical granting entities for your employers to support your art department.

So, who gets to the top here? Who finally makes it to the promise land as a Professor at a famous research university? Is it the best of the best, as the system intends? Or are we filtering for the people who are most willing to put up with abuse from their superiors? Are we simply reaching into the ranks to pull out the most subservient? Do you get to the top by being able to stand the longest amount of time at the very bottom? I'll come back to this thought a little later.

Chapter 2: Big pharma

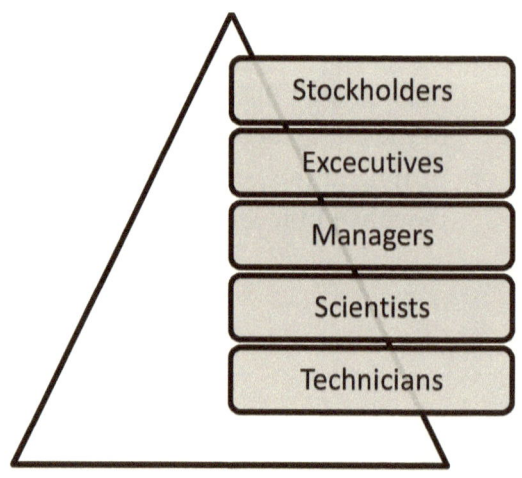

$500,000,000.00. Five hundred million dollars. This is the sum that most experts agree is necessary to develop a new drug, get it clinical trials and finally bring it to market. Whether we're talking antibiotics, chemotherapeutics, or stem cell therapies, all new treatments need to go through the following steps.

1.) **Development.** Someone needs to identify this new treatment. Currently, these new agents and treatment regiments come from basic research studies. Most new drugs are coming from high volume screens in which thousands of compounds are tested on bacteria, yeast, or cancer cells derived from a specific tumor. In this stage, thousands of compounds are narrowed down to a few dozen that show promise in this artificial system.

2.) **Animal Testing.** Typically these few dozen agents begin with treating mice that have been implanted with a specific tumor, are bred to have a genetic defect, or are infected with the disease of interest. The animals are treated with the drugs under study to determine if the agent is toxic to the animal and if the agent can actually improve the condition the mouse is now suffering from. A mouse used in this type of screening can cost anywhere from a few dozen to a few hundred dollars, depending on the lab and the conditions of the infirmity. Initial screens may involve only a small cohort of animals, maybe only a dozen. If the treatment actually shows some promise, the agent may eventually be tested on hundreds of different animal models. If the agent shows promise, but is damaging to the animal, the drug may be chemically modified before it is tested again. If it shows too many complications and not enough promise, the treatment is typically dropped.

3.) **Clinical trials.** There are multiple stages of clinical trials. Each stage is performed with human volunteers who are commonly paid for their participation on a sliding scale determined by how much time is required for their participation. For studies requiring weeks of 24 hour observation, I have heard of participants being paid as much as $15,000. During this study as many variables are eliminated as possible. All participants have the same diet and are often required to completely eat all of their meals, sleep the same number of hours and have similar amounts of physical activity.

Phase 0 clinical trials are often small groups who are given extremely low doses of the drug and the fate of the drug is monitored in their blood stream. Important variables are how much of the drug is broken down, as well as what is produced when the drug is broken down. For example, if human metabolism breaks down a drug to form a toxic by-product such as cyanide the drug can be scrapped at this point before people are ever dosed with an amount of the drug that might actually do harm.

Phase 1 trials are typically a larger group, often as many as 100. During this trial, participants are typically given increasingly higher doses of the drug over a period of time to determine the potential side effects of this treatment. These trials almost always require 24 hour observation by independent clinical nurses and physicians who have nothing to directly gain from the success or failure of the trial.

In **Phase 2** trials, the researchers actually try to determine if the drug works in humans. Volunteers are recruited who have a particular disease. For example, if this chemotherapy agent is thought to work against a particular form of cancer, oncology centers will specifically look for patients with this cancer that haven't had luck with other treatment options.

Phase 3 trials attempt to determine if this new treatment is any better than the treatments that are already available. What is the advantage of this new treatment over the ones that we already have and we already know is safe?

In some cases, phase 4 and 5 trials are necessary to determine the long term effects of this treatment plan. Whether they are necessary or not, it is easy to see where massive costs are accrued during this process. Hundreds, sometimes thousands of people, must be tested. Physicians and medical personnel must be available around the clock to monitor participants for side effects. What happens if a drug gets to phase 3 trials and then fails? Then the new treatment accrued all of these costs for nothing. You can monitor the stocks of big companies during clinical trials and see how they go through sharp increases in value as each phase is successfully navigated. More often than not, you will find a massive sell-off that occurred within a few days of the failure of the agent in phase 3 or 4. For example, Curis pharmaceutical stock fell over 40% in one day in the June of 2010 after experimental drug 0449 didn't succeed in clinical trials.

For the rare drug or treatment that does succeed, the company must now figure out a way to recoup its costs, not only for this drug, but also for all the drugs preceding it that failed. And this is where problems arise.

Nearly every expert on bacteria in the world agrees that at some point in the near future, all the antibiotics on earth are going to be pretty much useless. Every few weeks I hear about a new 'super-strain' of some pathogenic bacteria that is immune to nearly every antibiotic on earth. At first, these strains received lots of media attention and threatening acronyms, such as MRSA, which is short for methicillin resistant *Staph aureus*. MRSA has received the most attention in the U.S., as it has been contracted by a number of young athletes through minor injuries. If this disease can start as minor turf burn on someone as healthy as a football player and kill him a few short days later, it is definitely something to be concerned about for the rest of us who are nowhere near as healthy or conditioned. The occurrence of MRSA is so common these days that it no longer makes the nightly news. Even more frightening is MRSA's close relative VRSA which is immune to vancomycin, the one drug that MRSA is sometimes susceptible to. Only surgically removing the infected tissue is effective in stopping the spread of this disease.

There is one thing that I find more frightening than these new super bugs - the fact that there are no new antibiotics on the way. That's right. Virtually no new antibiotics have entered clinical trials in the last 10 years. The reason for this is very simple. How much do antibiotics cost? I know that a department store pharmacy near my home advertises several antibiotics on its $4 prescription list. The other problem is that you only take one prescription of an antibiotic. Your doctor prescribes you one bottle and you take it and you're better. Even if the antibiotic is an expensive new name brand, it never costs much more than $100. How many people need to contract this bacterial infection for the pharmaceutical company to make a profit on its drug? More than 5 million people would have to contract this disease and exclusively use this new antibiotic for treatment. Until these super-strains begin killing people by the tens of thousands, we won't see antibiotics appear to combat them. Due to the amount of time that is required for a drug to proceed through development and clinical trials it is likely that new drugs won't reach your pharmacy until the death toll has reached unprecedented levels.

The high cost of bringing treatments to market is also affecting the promising field of stem cell treatment. Although government funding has allowed the development of dozens of new stem cell lines that are derived from adult human cells, the field of stem cell treatment effectively halted recently. In the first clinical trials of using cultured stem cells to cure a disease, the single treatment outcome was so positive that the trials were halted.

I was sitting in the audience at the world's largest meeting on stem cells in 2009 when one of the most prominent researchers in the field unveiled this finding. During the collective gasp of the audience as we considered the implications he walked off of the stage and out of the conference. Why would they halt the development of a treatment that was so promising? A single treatment has the same problem as the new antibiotic does; how do we recoup our costs if the patient only receives one treatment? In order to make a profit, the company would have to charge $1 million dollars for the treatment of each patient, a cost that no insurance company in the world would agree to pay.

In order to combat this problem several labs have been working on the development of stem cell lines that are dependent on specific chemicals to survive. The hope is that big companies would be interested in developing stem cell treatments if the recipients of the stem cells are dependent for the rest of their lives on the expensive drug they sell that keep those cells alive. Even though I understand the requirement of a company to make profit, the whole concept makes me nauseous.

These are just two examples of the difficulties that arise when drug development decisions are ultimately made by corporate executives who must make decisions based solely on the cost of development versus the potential profits of the drug.

In order to lower the costs of drug development, one strategy companies have employed recently has been to purchase agents developed by the government. Occasionally a new drug is invented or discovered by a small government or academic lab that is so promising that the government will pay for the animal testing and clinical trials for this treatment. A few years ago, a small California-based company developed one such agent. Due to the costs of developing the agent, the company asked the government for assistance with the testing and trials. One government research institute agreed and spent more than 5 years developing this agent, which eventually squeaked through all trial phases and was approved for use in humans. Due to either a poorly executed legal agreement, or simply due to the fact that the administration at this agency underestimated the human greed, this new drug is available to very few patients. This is due to the fact that the new chemotherapy drug went on the market at the cost of $13,000 per dose. In 2010 the average 1 year treatment with this drug cost approximately $200,000. The distributor of this medication has recorded record 9-figure profits ever since and the majority of the development costs of this agent fell on the shoulders of U.S. taxpayers.

Lawsuits

Another deterrent in the development of new treatments are lawsuits. As I mentioned in the introduction, the majority of cancer treatments in use today were first implemented in the 1950s. Radiation and the use of DNA damaging chemotherapy agents are still the most common ways of treating almost every type of cancer, today they are simply more fine-tuned. Both of these treatments work in the same way, by damaging all the cells in your body.

One way that cancer cells differ from other cells in your body is that cancer cells can't stop dividing. Generally, if a normal cell is damaged, especially in its DNA, it will stop dividing and will not resume growth or cell division until the damage has been repaired. Radiation and most chemotherapy drugs damage the DNA in every cell in your body to about the same level. While most normal cells stop dividing and go about repairing the damage, cancer cells keep on dividing. This damage only multiplies with further cell divisions and (if all goes well) the cancer cells die. Many of the side effects of radiation and chemotherapy are the result of fast dividing cells, such as the ones in your gastrointestinal tract, dying from the treatment because, like cancer cells, they can't stop dividing. The symptoms subside when these normal cells are replaced by your body's natural reserves of stem cells.

Every time I watch network television I see commercials telling me about class-action lawsuits that are being waged against pharmaceutical companies. These lawsuits are being waged on the behalf of patients who have been prescribed recently-developed medications and who have had side effects from these treatments.

Stop for a second and imagine the side effects that you know about chemotherapy and radiation. Severe nausea, hair loss, muscle weakness for weeks or months, immune system suppression, and so on. If these treatments were developed by a pharmaceutical company in the 1990s, would this company have survived the onslaught of lawsuits to even be in business today? It is a common opinion among pharmacologists that many, if not most, common medications, even over the counter ones, we use in the U.S. would never be used if they were invented today.

What company would even consider developing the next chemotherapy agent that had side effects anywhere near as severe as those of the old drugs?

Chapter 3: Government labs

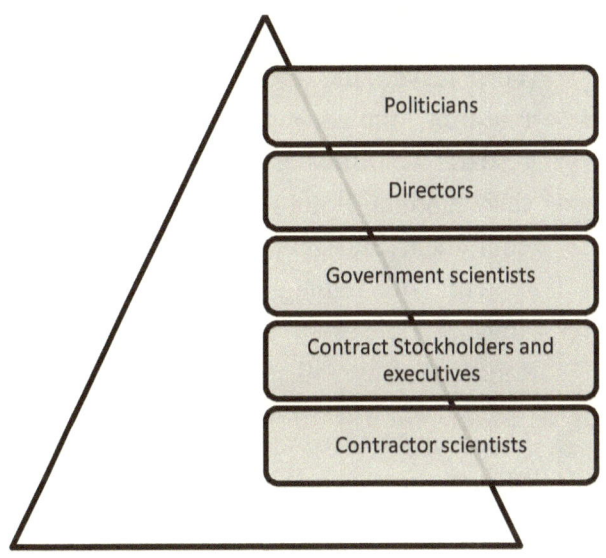

Researchers in academic labs are under extremely high levels of stress due to their workloads throughout their career and by the sheer bulk of the student loans they incur to obtain their degrees. On top of that, the majority of the money they are given to perform their research is subverted to other goals. It is unlikely that with this limited time, energy and resources that anyone from the academic ranks will have the ability in the near future to propel us toward the next advancement in curing cancer. Big pharma has fewer of these constraints, but unless the next cancer treatment can somehow evade rigorous clinical trials or is guaranteed to pay big bucks, and has virtually no side effects, they aren't going to pursue it.

This leaves the final stronghold for biomedical research, the government sector. Government research facilities have the following advantages: few funding limitations, plenty of resources for equipment and manpower, and significantly less danger of damaging lawsuits. With these advantages, surely the next big breakthrough in cancer therapy will come from this sector.

Government research is generally provided by two distinct entities, government employees and government contractors. Contractors work directly for corporations that are under contract from the government to provide services such as research. These contracts are typically 5 – 10 years long, giving the employees job security during this time. When the contract is up, however, other companies may submit rival bids to the current one and the best deal is taken by the government. If you are an employee of the old company, you are out of a job and are left hoping that the new contract holder is interested in your services. On top of this, individual contractors may lose their positions at any time, as the contracting company has the same freedom to lay-off or discharge employees as any other company, a leisure that is not shared by the federal government. A part-time occupation of contractors, especially near the end of a contract, is attempting to find a more stable job, hopefully one as a full government employee. In exchange for this level of uncertainty, contract employees typically make more money than a government employee that holds the same position. Contractors also have more defined vacation and sick leave plans with guaranteed vacation time even for postdocs.

One reason the government uses contractors for research is because no presidential administration wants to admit that the government became larger under their watch. Contractors are hired in order to keep the official numbers low, despite the increase in research demands. Every year more contractors are hired for central government agencies and the administration can truthfully claim that these agencies did not become larger during their tenure. In order to hire a contract researcher you must employee a contract company. This company will be responsible for the employee's health plan, payroll, retirement plan, *et cetera*. In order to provide these services, the contract company must charge fees well above the salary of the contract employee. These fees are typically equivalent to the salary of that employee, making it cost more than twice as much to employ that researcher over an equivalent government scientist.

The tradeoff for making a less money is that government positions are considerably more stable. Tenured government employees generally enjoy job stability on a level equivalent to their counterparts in academia. Unlike contract postdocs, most government postdocs have no set hours and no guarantees that they can take sick time or vacation time. Typically, however, the environment is less conducive to abuse by data hungry supervisors than the academic system. The pay is also better than in the academic system. As I mentioned earlier, the NIH pays their postdocs considerably more than they recommend that other labs pay their postdocs. Within the NIH a first year postdoc will begin with a salary around $45K. During austerity plans such as the one put in place in 2010, the salaries of all government employees, including postdocs, are frozen and do not increase at the guaranteed rate specified in their contracts. This can be a particular challenge for those with large student loan debts due to the graduate repayment plan. This plan is structured so that student loan payments increase over time to match the expected increases in the postdoc's salary. While austerity plans freeze the government postdoc salaries, the plans do not freeze the increase in the student loan payments.

One interesting facet of government research is in the budgeting of money within a laboratory. Due to the fact that government agencies often don't actually know how much funding they will receive from the federal budget until near the end of the fiscal year, the last few months are often very hectic. Typically, the final operating budget for each lab will be received by the lab manager around July or August, with the fiscal year ending the first day of October. If the lab has spent more money than it was allotted due to poor budgeting the manager looks for funding from senior management to shore up the difference. In this situation, the lab manager often starts looking for a new position. Another challenge arises when the lab has not spent enough money. I have been to countless meetings in my career where an obviously exhausted senior investigator has said something like "I've been up all night trying to spend as much money as possible, but we still have $200,000 and only 3 weeks to spend it." Generally, I can come up with a few purchases that will make life easier around the lab or improve the quality of my research, but the first thing I think is that I would like to have some of my taxes back. I have NEVER been in a meeting where the senior investigator or lab manager says "we spent far less than we were budgeted, good job everyone, we're going to give it back to the taxpayers." During these spending frenzies I wonder if every lab with a surplus gave it back if it would make a difference in this huge deficit we're sitting in.

In most government facilities there are old offices or storage rooms that are completely full of previously purchased, but unopened, supplies. I once saw with a sign beside the door that said "Excess budget purchases, 2005." While I didn't get to see inside the door, I was told that there were approximately 40,000 15 milliliter conical tubes that were purchased by a now-retired scientist as her last effort to use up all the money in her budget. This frenzy is due to one shared fear among all scientists receiving government funds – if you don't use all the money, next year they will cut your budget. In my time in government funded research, I am not aware of this happening to my labs, but the rumor persists. The majority of researchers believe that it would be much better to purchase supplies that they might not need than to be caught the following year with a desperate need for something they won't be able to buy.

Despite the strange use of budgeting, the government system looks like the best of the three research realms. Highly motivated contractors who badly want to keep their jobs work hand-in-hand with government employees who have more stable positions. In exchange for stability, contractors make a little more money, but during fiscal cutbacks the research can continue due to the fact that the government employees still have their jobs. They just have to do a lot more work now that the contractors are unemployed.

At first, this system worked really well, as you would expect it should. In the 1960s and 1970s, these large government facilities aided in rolling out several new chemotherapies and identified a number of viable drug targets. Then the unthinkable happened. Two labs at the same facility published papers at the same time with completely opposite results. One publication in a prestigious journal clearly showed that a new chemotherapy drug worked through one pathway and should progress to human testing. The second lab showed that the drug worked through a completely different pathway and that the drug should immediately be dropped from further study. To make matters worse, the heads of both labs were both well respected and both publications appeared in very high ranking journals. To make this clear, conflicting studies happen all the time, especially on promising chemotherapy drugs that dozens of labs are studying at once. In this case, the response from the scientific community was unfairly harsh and both labs and the large institution were openly derided in many publications and at many major scientific conferences.

The black eye that effectively resulted from these studies caused a complete restructuring of this government entity. A strict hierarchy was put into place with a number of prestigious physicians recruited from academic and pharmaceutical labs placed at the top of the system. An immediate directive was issued that all scientific results performed by all labs within this government entity had to be approved by senior management before they could be released to the public. The first problem with this setup was that just one of the facilities operated by this entity employed nearly 5,000 people. The researchers at this facility prepare hundreds of papers a year for publication. An immediate backlog appeared in which taxpayer funded research on important new chemotherapies may sit for years before they could reach the scientific and medical communities.

In medical research, prominence typically correlates with the age of the scientist. Older scientists are generally better known and have had more time to succeed than younger scientists. Only recently have we seen scientists begin to rise from the ranks of groups such as women and minorities. As a result, when searching for leaders to run the government's largest and most well-funded cancer research center, they had a small group to pick from, consisting primarily of white male physicians who graduated from the premier Ivy League institution between 1965 and 1975.

The ethnic background of these men and the school they all graduated from is fundamentally unimportant, I just put those facts in there because they are true and it helps to give an idea of just who I'm talking about. Now, you learn a lot in medical school. You study anatomy, biology, chemistry, and biochemistry, along with other subjects. With the obvious exception of anatomy, all of these subjects have progressed more since 1975 than they have in the thousand years prior. These days it's almost impossible for one person to be fluent in every technology in even one of these fields, let alone all of them. As a result, the heads of this institution are constantly required to learn about new technologies and new techniques in order to review the work of the thousands of researchers under them.

During my time working at this facility I had to deliver results of my research to these men, in person, a number of times. The technologies I use in my work have been in use continuously for the last 10 to 15 years and the development of these techniques have resulted in several Nobel Prizes. Despite these facts, my supervisor would spend at least 2 days prior to my talks 'dumbing down' my research to be digestible by our superiors.

Unfortunately, the majority of the discussion time after my presentations was spent explaining how these techniques work in the broadest terms possible. Despite these preparations we knew that they had missed the true significance of our work and that our publications would be pushed further down the pile. To be clear, this wasn't because of intellectual short-comings of the senior administration of this institution. It is because it is simply impossible for one person to keep up with all of the research occurring, and technology in use, at an institution of that size. The refusal of these men to relinquish any amount of authority to reviewers who are more qualified to guide specific types of research only serves to harm the individual labs and the institution.

A second problem exists here, of course. There are a number of clichés about power that we all know, particularly about the corruption of power. Imagine what happens when a group of people who graduate from the same school at the same time and work in the same field are given power over nearly every person in their field of study. The resulting corruption is inevitable, as is the continuing thirst for power. This case is no exception.

Within a few years, the senior administration was no longer content with simply approving research for release to the public; they also wanted control over every study performed by every cancer researcher in the country. Control over the academic labs was easy, as the largest source of funding for cancer research in the world, they could simply reject grant applications that they didn't like and provide funding to people and projects that they did like.

Suddenly we saw an even higher percentage of grant applications at certain schools (one school in particular) being approved and the numbers aren't even close. Coincidentally, these schools also happen to be the *alma maters* of the same administrators. It is even easier to guess what research they liked to approve. If you had the choice, would you fund research that you were comfortable with, that you could easily understand, or research that you had trouble grasping? It quickly became apparent that if you were using traditional scientific techniques then you had a much better chance of being funded. Unfortunately, these are the same techniques that have yet to improve the efficacy of cancer treatment; nonetheless these are the studies with the highest likelihood of being funded.

Implementing this same approach within the government agency proved to be slightly more difficult. Government employees within this institution had been used to working nearly independently on their research, often for decades and resisted increased control over their budgets and their research goals. The recent recession gave these men the power they needed. With the exception of the military research labs, nearly all government research facilities were told to cut their spending in 2011 by 10-20%. Most entities responded by telling principal investigators to cut their budgets by the appropriate percentage and left the details up to each lab. One government entity responded by cutting nearly all of their contractor support staff. The entity responsible for cancer research had a different idea.

In the summer of 2011, the heads of this institute asked for every lab to submit a list of research projects that they planned to perform during the following year. Despite the amount of progress that had been made on this study, or whether it had been previously approved, if it was not approved by this new panel then the work must stop immediately. In this way, the men at the top had complete control over every study performed at their institution. Within two months of the announcement, the two most famous researchers at this institution were gone. The first left his lab for a purported multi-million dollar contract with a pharmaceutical company.

The second researcher to leave is the world's premier expert on Alveolar Soft Part Sarcoma (ASPS); we'll call him Dr. D. A diagnosis of ASPS is essentially a death sentence due to the fact that the tumors formed are slow growing and are resistant to virtually all forms of cancer treatments, including chemotherapy and radiation. The only treatment available is multiple surgeries to remove the growing tumors. Since they tend to grow slowly, people suffering from this condition end up having an operation every few years to remove the tumors until the combination of damage from the surgeries and the tumor growth takes the patient's life. Dr. D's lab had been focused on studying ASPS since his child was diagnosed with the condition decades earlier, when he dropped everything and began studying this mysterious condition.

The results of Dr. D's efforts were a new mutant mouse strain that suffered from ASPS. New chemotherapy agents and combinations of different treatments could be tested on these mice in order to find drugs that work against ASPS. Despite his success in this field and the fact that Dr. D had been working at the institution since he had completed his Ph.D., his funding was cut and he was pressured into retiring before he felt his work on this disease was done.

Around that same time, a study in my lab on a promising chemotherapy drug was also halted. The study was 90% completed and needed a few weeks of work before it could be written up for publication but was not approved to continue. Work stopped on this project even though the supplies were already purchased and the work was being performed by completely free labor in the form of a graduate student from Europe. The completion of this project was the final chapter of his thesis and the result of months of volunteer labor that he had performed in our lab. Despite multiple pleas from this student and the head of our department for the senior administration to think logically, or sympathetically, the project was scrapped.

Unfortunately, even projects allowed to continue under this new approval system weren't safe. Monthly meetings were scheduled for groups to demonstrate their progress on the approved projects. It wasn't uncommon for an approved project to be cut in front of everyone with the explanation such as, "we didn't understand what the project was about until now."

The projects that did receive funding, received lots of it. And you could always tell what project would receive the money. Does the project use outdated technology that has been shown not to work? Does it deal with failed chemotherapy agents once championed by a member of the senior administration? Does it involve collaboration with one of their personal laboratories? If so, then praise and money will be heaped upon the researcher and their laboratory.

While the men I've described are the senior directors of this institution, it is worth noting that the actual Head of the institution was appointed for the task by our most recent president. This particular man was instrumental in helping to develop our early understanding of cancer. For his years of service he was even awarded a Nobel Prize for a discovery one of his technicians made in his laboratory. Since that time he has primarily withdrawn from science and has spent his time in the world of politics, even publishing a very nice book on the subject a few years ago. As a political appointee he obviously has to answer for the actions of the institution to members of Congress, not to mention the President himself. Politicians also decide the annual budget that is allotted for this institution, as well as how and when new hires are made. With all of this political pressure surrounding the institution, what would happen if someone near the top messed up? Would the mistake and the details of this mistake be openly aired and the problem worked out? Or would the mistake simply disappear forever?

Why We Haven't Cured Cancer

A few years ago a senior researcher at a remote facility operated by the institution began a multi-million dollar study to look closely at the DNA of multiple cancer cell lines. Most of this work was to be performed by different private companies and the head researcher's primary tasks were to design the experiments, distribute the samples and fees to the biotech companies, and evaluate the results. Apparently, very little new information came from this set of experiments, something that commonly occurs in science, and the results were never released. Following this failure, the researcher took a job with a private biotech company on the other side of the globe. Even though the experiments were purported to be a failure, some researchers at the institution were curious to see the data generated in order to compare it with their own data. Surprisingly, no one could find these results. In fact, upon further investigation no one could find records of the samples being sent out or exactly what companies received this money. By the time someone started to realize that millions of dollars and a senior researcher were gone, she had been gone for years. If it had been a few months, I'm sure the FBI would have been contacted and she would be in prison somewhere. Unfortunately, it had been years. Although this discovery would not cost the new institution Head his position, it would definitely cost members of the senior administration their jobs. These revelations would likely cause a negative impact on the budget and standing of the institution, particularly after the details of the case were revealed in court. In order to protect their positions, the senior management silenced this case and the researcher continues to enjoy her time on the beach somewhere.

Recently, a completely new class of chemotherapy agents has come into view on the world stage. These drugs are able to inhibit the ability of cancer cells to repair their DNA, while doing little to harm normal cells. For the sake of brevity, I'll call them DNArIs (short for DNA repair inhibitors). They have become such big business that a professor who invented one of the first of these drugs sold the rights for it to a pharmaceutical company for a sum thought to be nearly $300 million. This drug was the first of this new class to go into clinical trials, where it failed completely, shocking the entire scientific community. Several other drugs in this class that were slated to begin clinical trials were immediately halted.

In 2010 I attended a large meeting where the drug was described to dozens of government labs and the goal was set to figure out why the drug didn't work as expected. The meeting was organized by a new director at our facility, a rising star in the cancer research community, Dr. E., who also happened to be the first female director at this institution. As directed, our lab and many others dropped nearly all of our other work to pursue this compound. Within a week it was clear to us that something fishy was happening. This drug didn't seem to function the same way as the other DNArIs. After a month we sat down and decided to drop the hypothesis that the drug was a DNArI completely. We had solid proof that this drug did not work in anywhere near the same way as reported, and that it didn't even seem to have an effect on DNA at all. Within another month we had our answer. This drug was not a DNArI; it was a generic toxin that just happened to trigger a DNA repair protein in lab rats before it destroyed the other proteins in the body. In all, we were able to detect nearly 1,000 human proteins that this drug attached to and inactivated, functioning as one of the most unspecific poisons in medical history.

Without question, our lab was considered one of the single best in the institution. This was probably due to the unique management plan we had in place. The lab was operated by two senior scientists who shared an obsession with new scientific technology. They are two of the most dedicated researchers I have ever met, with the vast majority of their free time devoted to reading the literature and attending seminars on new technologies. As a result of this and a long history of success, we had both the interest in, and the funds to secure, the most cutting edge technology available. In order to run this technology, the lab was required to recruit young researchers from other labs successful enough to have access to these devices.

Dozens of labs began work with this new agent at the same time. It was pretty obvious that whoever solved this riddle would immediately gain favor with the new director. As such, we were sworn to complete secrecy on this (and most other) projects. Here is the problem. We shared our floor with two other labs that also began work on this agent. As I mentioned, we realized within weeks that the drug didn't do anything remotely similar to what it was purported to do. A few months later, we had solved the mechanism of action of this agent. Since we shared a break room and common area with the other labs, we all knew that the other two labs were still working under the incorrect premise that the drug was a DNArI even months after we had solved the drug. With the work finished, the other labs – at least 12 of them were essentially working on a project that was already completed. How many tax payer dollars would have been saved, or diverted to better uses, if we had communicated our findings with the other lab directors and had been working together, rather than competing against each other?

With our data solidly in hand and replicated numerous times we asked for an audience with our new director in order to present these findings. Obviously, she was skeptical at first, we were suggesting that a drug thought to be worth billions was actually a sham and a poison. As we stacked the results of clear experiments one after another on her desk, she realized that we were right. She asked us to give this presentation to the senior administration in a closed door meeting.

Every member of the senior administration attended this meeting. The only notable absence was that of Dr. E. Rather than being allowed to present our data, the deputy director told us to stop all work on this drug and to never mention it to anyone. He had received the results of our study from Dr. E. and they knew what we had to say. He also knew that the institute had given this poison to hundreds of human volunteers during the clinical trials on the mistaken belief that the drug did what they were told it would do. Our findings would only embarrass the institution and endanger their beloved positions atop the scientific community. Meanwhile, researchers at another clinic were continuing to perform clinical trials with this poison and our nondisclosure agreements ensured that we would be ruined if we said a word of this to anyone. On a more personal note, if we had published this study, it would have been a groundbreaking achievement for our lab, practically ensuring that our hard-working postdocs would achieve the success that they earned. As a direct result of the suppression of this data I and two other members of our laboratory handed in our resignations.

In summary, the world's largest government entity devoted to cancer research takes in approximately $5 billion dollars a year in U.S. taxpayer dollars. Some of this money is dedicated to academic labs, with the majority of the money going to the *alma maters* of the senior administrators of this institution. The money that is retained is currently used to fund outdated research on drugs that have been shown to be ineffective in cancer treatment or in studying promising new agents with slow, outdated technology that the administration is comfortable with. The results of this work are withheld from the scientific and medical community for political reasons, even when it is endangering the lives of clinical testing volunteers.

Footnote: During the fall of 2011, while placing the finished touches on this text, a research study performed at a small college finally revealed the true nature of this drug we were tasked with studying. The results matched ours exactly. These results were published in a journal that I had never previously heard of. I wonder if the results were considered too controversial for publication by the more well-known companies. It is also possible that the lab that made this discovery couldn't afford to publish their results in the more well-known journals (more on this later). In any case, I'm sure that these results will be questioned, and ultimately substantiated by other labs.

When the true nature of this compound is accepted by the scientific community, this drug will finally be removed from clinical testing facilities and deposited in hazardous waste containers where it belongs.

Section 2: Where Does the Money Go?

In the following sections we'll take a look at where the money provided by the government to do research is actually going. We've already seen that in most cases the majority of money given in the form of government grants for academic research goes to support other causes rather than actual research. The remaining amount is actually used for purposes it was meant for such as researcher salaries, supplies and equipment, and the publishing and access to scientific data.

Chapter 4: Scientific equipment and supply companies

This chapter must merely deal with the services provided by supply and equipment companies, as I've never worked for one and really don't know what the employment conditions are like at their facilities. The following table contains the description and prices of 6 items that I obtained from the website of a major scientific supply company where I commonly place orders.

Product	Price
6% Sodium hypochlorite(1L)	$36.04
6% Sodium hypochlorite (4L)	$80.57
Aluminum foil standard gauge 12 in. x 200 ft.	$67.84
13 Gallon tall kitchen trash bags (100 pk)	$74.32
16 oz. empty spray bottles (6 pk)	$66.53
Fine tip permanent markers (10 pk)	$47.53

Does 6% sodium hypochlorite sound familiar? It should. Its more common name is bleach. And 6% bleach is roughly the same concentration that you find in your neighborhood grocery store. At our local union operated grocery store, name brand bleach runs $2.99 for roughly 3.8 liters (1 gallon) and that actually seems a little high to me. Compare this to the $80.57 for 4 liters as shown in the table. My grocery store certainly beats ordering it from the company I took this price table from. The one thing that is nice to see is that you do get a discount for purchasing larger amounts, such as the steep price drop from buying one 4L bottle of bleach, rather than four 1L bottles.

Bleach isn't an anomaly, either. At this same company's website, a 200 foot roll of 12 inch wide, standard gauge aluminum foil will run you $67; try comparing this to the price at your local grocery store. You probably don't buy your trash bags in packages of 100, but I certainly wouldn't buy any size box of trash bags for $74, especially not for the exact same brand and size that we use in my home. I could fill this chapter with other examples, but I think you get the point; if you used these values on the "Price is Right" game show, you'll almost certainly go home empty-handed (and your fellow contestants may question your sanity). However, these are the standard prices that we pay for lab supplies. Admittedly, for these common items many labs will send a technician, a couple of times a year, to the grocery store with a lab credit card, but I want to stop here and consider the implications.

On these common items we can easily see a 10 to 30 fold markup over normal commercial suppliers. What is the markup on items that we can't see? 100-fold? When I buy a piece of equipment for $16,000, did it cost $160 to build, or even less?

Why We Haven't Cured Cancer

Years ago an acquaintance of mine started his own lab in his back yard in order to work on environmentally friendly alternatives to common lab supplies. He made a surprising amount of his lab equipment by hand. A centrifuge is a common device in all research labs. They consist of three parts, a rotor to place samples in, a motor that spins the rotor, and a control unit for selecting the speed of the motor. Rather than purchasing a standard centrifuge for anywhere between $600 and $4000, he purchased a rotor and attached it to the top of a blender. While the $60 he spent on this device did not give him the speed or control options of a top level centrifuge, it did vastly exceed the capabilities of a base model centrifuge, a device that would have cost him at least 10 times more. While this obviously is not a viable solution for most labs, it worked out well for my friend who patented dozens of his alternative lab supplies that are marketed by companies around the world.

We'll probably never know the real market value of the equipment we are purchasing. What we do know, however, is that the current system is working pretty well. The following chart is a snapshot of the stock prices of the scientific supply company in question on January 1st for the last ten years (rounded to the nearest dollar).

Why We Haven't Cured Cancer

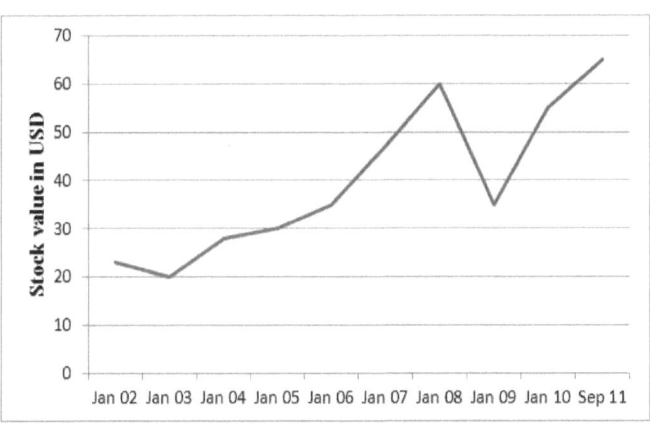

From this snapshot, it looks like business is going pretty well. With the exception of a brief drop off at the beginning of 2009, it seems like a period of fantastic growth. That drop-off, by the way, was due to this company purchasing one of its struggling competitors. Just for comparison's sake, the following figure is a graph of the stock prices of one of the world's largest retailers over the exact same time period.

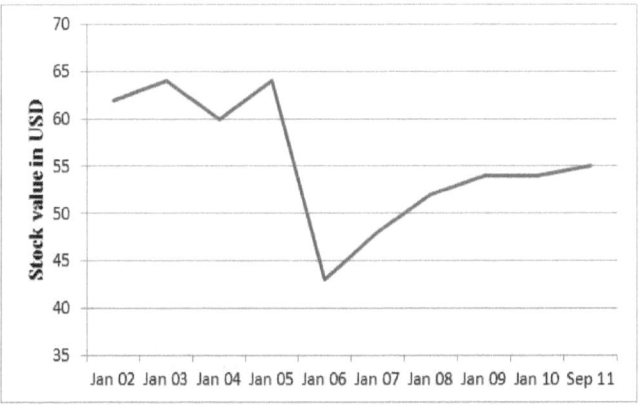

For some reason the stock prices of this retailer seem very different from that of our scientific supplier. In fact, business doesn't seem to be doing very well at all, especially around the middle of the graph. I'm no expert in economics, but I have a feeling that this downturn may have had something to do with the global recession.

In summary, if you purchase products from a scientific supply company that you could easily obtain from a normal commercial retailer, you should expect to pay about ten to twenty times more at the supply company. This business model works so well that in the middle of the second largest financial downturn in United States history, you can still afford to purchase one of your competitors and it will take you about 2 years during this recession before you are back to making record profits.

This begs the question: Just what are these companies doing to justify these mind-boggling fees and unprecedented financial security? Honestly, I can't answer this question with any statistical evidence, but I do have a few anecdotes that could help you get an idea.

When I was in graduate school, I really wanted to automate a complex and annoying process for identifying and quantifying a specific type of molecule produced by some cancer cells. I had the device that would separate these molecules connected to the analyzer that would identify them. All I needed in the middle was a detector that could quantify them for me. With this process streamlined, I would be able to study twice as many cancer lines in the same amount of time and publish this method for other labs to use. I contacted a sales representative who worked for the company that built, serviced, and sold us all of this equipment and received a quote of $10,000 for the detector I needed for this project

In my spare time I wrote 4 grants to try and raise money for this detector. I received money for two of these grants and my advisor saved some money when one of my fellow graduate students dropped out of our program. With these funds and the university's bulk discount we were able to purchase the detector. Six months later, the detector arrived. (I now know that 6 months to receive your order on pieces of equipment such as this one is considered pretty good service.) The installation technician showed up two weeks later and he attempted to install the detector. He failed. Unfortunately, the sales representative wasn't nearly as familiar with our software package as he had claimed and he was unaware that this device was not compatible with the software running our separator and analyzer. Never fear, though! We could purchase the compatible software package for the meager sum of $7,000. The thought of raising even more money for this project was, unfortunately, completely out of the question.

To this day, as far as I know, that detector still sits in a box in a supply closet in my old advisor's lab. Of course we couldn't return the device; it had been 'installed' by their technician. I attempted to write a software patch to make the detector compatible with our current equipment, but it never really worked to its full capacity. We eventually abandoned it and the project. Can you imagine the outrage if a big budget retailer sold computer peripheral devices without the software necessary to operate that device? What if you brought hardware home you bought for your PC and found that it only worked on a Mac and the store refused to take a return? A normal retailer that treated their customers in such a way would soon find themselves out of business. Why can a manufacturer of scientific equipment afford to operate in such a way?

As a side note, I'd like you to know that I have gotten some measure of revenge on the company that sold this detector. A major component of my career has been starting up new bioanalytical labs at academic, government, and private research facilities. As a consequence, my opinions on equipment tend to be taken very seriously. I'll just say that I'm not so quick to recommend hardware made by a certain manufacturer, and that $10,000 detector has probably cost them a few hundred times more than that in potential sales with which I have been involved.

Shortly after the congressional elections in 2010 a number of disagreements over the federal budget left all government labs unable to spend money for short periods of time. During one of these periods I was forced to contact technical support on one of our analytical devices. Although the equipment had not been used, it sat in a box pending permission from the government to install for so long that the 1 year warranty expired (most manufacturer's begin your warranty from the date of installation, just not this company). While talking to them about the repair, I mentioned that I couldn't currently purchase the small fitting that had deteriorated during storage, (it cost around $450) but if they would send me one so that I could begin working with the device I could easily pay them back after the spending freeze was lifted. Despite the fact that this $450 part was all that was stopping the operation of a $1 million analytical device, I never heard from that service representative again. Fortunately I was able to claim, quite truthfully, that this part was of essential to my research and the government released enough money to make this purchase. However, this is another company that will never receive my business again.

So the prices are inflated beyond any rational amount, and the service is at least not uncommonly poor. Why do we buy from these companies? The answer, unfortunately, is because we have to. The agencies that issue research funds have regulations on where you can purchase equipment and scientific supplies. During my postdoc I ordered a synthetic material, on which to do my dissections. A month after I placed the order I received the wrong product. When speaking to customer service about this product I mentioned that I'd just order it from Amazon (where it was one-tenth the price and I knew I would receive the order both correctly and punctually). The conversation was relayed to my supervisors and I was reprimanded for even considering purchasing the material from such a vendor.

Firmly established in my career years later and I still don't know where these rules are made, or who makes them. I do know that when writing your results for publication there is a section for materials and methods, where most authors describe the procedure and where they obtain their equipment and supplies. Perhaps the concern is that we would be scorned, or our papers rejected, if the editors and reviewers saw that we bought our supplies at a lower price than they did. I understand the importance of using high quality supplies for scientific research. Most reagents are scrutinized by multiple rounds of quality control and assurance protocols. I wouldn't dream of reporting a result from an experiment that I obtained using hydrochloric acid from the hardware store since the impurities, and how they affect my experiment, are completely unknown. I do not, however, believe that the trash bags I use in my office will adversely affect my results, especially when they are identical to the ones I use in my kitchen at home.

Chapter 5: Publishing

Peer-Reviewed Journal Articles

Publishing research is critical for scientific advancement. No important research begins without understanding what has been done previously. Every major advancement in history started with one person reading another person's findings and either explaining these findings, or taking the research one step further.

As I described in the previous sections, researchers in academia and government are required to publish summaries of their research in peer-reviewed journals in order to keep or further their careers. This chapter will explain how an experiment makes it from the researcher, into a journal, and finally into the hands of other scientists.

Step 1, Writing

This can be the easiest part of the process, but it is often the hardest. Everyone in a lab who contributed to a project sits down and generally the authors bring all the relevant data. The authors hash out the details such as the hypothesis, and what data best supports the conclusions of the paper. In my experience, this is often where the order of authorship is decided.

Ideal circumstances: everyone has a clear understanding of what they brought to the paper and how much they contributed to the study as a whole. In these circumstances everyone who contributed is present and you can easily decide who is first, second or third author.

A common problem during this process occurs when one contributor believes that his/her contribution to the project is substantially more valuable than the rest of the group considers this contribution. Many labs, for this reason, include every member of their lab on every publication and clearly assign the role of first author on this study before the research has actually started. The problem here, unfortunately, is that lab members who had nothing to do with this project will appear to be experts in the procedures and techniques used in this study when they have never participated in this study at all. When authorship is assigned in this way, supporting authors may be less motivated to contribute as much effort to this project. Another problem arises here when prior postdocs or graduate students in a lab see a publication after it has been published and claim, accurately or not, that they contributed to that study and were not acknowledged for their work. Situations like this have been the grounds of many, sometimes successful, lawsuits. Its common practice for labs to list any of their recent employees as authors who, again, may not have any experience with the methods employed in this study, but at least the lab avoids a lawsuit.

Step 2, Selecting an Appropriate Journal

Once you've written the bulk of the paper its time to select an appropriate journal. In every field there is an appropriate hierarchy. If your study is groundbreaking to the extent that it transcends your field and would be interesting for any person in any field of science then it goes into *Science, Nature,* or *The Proceedings of the National Academy of Science*. If it's groundbreaking for biology, then it goes into *Cell,* and if it's only groundbreaking for your field, then it goes into the highest ranked journal in your field. In order to tell where to publish your work, there are multiple organizations that rank the importance of academic journals, assigning them something called an impact factor. Every person and every journal has their favorite impact factor system. My favorite is the one that ranks the journals I've published in the highest. Likewise, every journal displays on their home page the ratings of the system that gives them the highest ranking. If you are unsure of the impact of your work you can send it to the highest journal first. If the editor and reviewers don't think your work is of the appropriate scale for their journal, you'll know within a day or two. You can then send it to the next highest journal, or if you're really lucky, the editor may suggest an appropriate place to publish your work.

Step 3, Submission and Peer Review

Once you've hammered out the paper and decided where to send it, you submit the research (in the appropriate format) along with supporting information to the journal of your choice. An editor is assigned to your paper and decides whether it would be an asset to this journal. If it is, they will send your work out to 2-4 researchers in the field who are qualified to evaluate your work. Some journals even allow you to recommend appropriate reviewers or to tell them the names of your mortal enemies so that they don't review (and reject) your work. You typically know within a few days if your work will be peer-reviewed and these reviews come back in a few weeks. The anonymous reviewers have to answer two main questions about your submission: Should it be accepted? And what is wrong with it? If your paper is to be rejected, the answers tend to be really short. Answers such as, "I don't believe this work is within the scope of this journal" and "further studies are necessary to complete this work" are common. If the reviewers agree to accept this work, the suggestions will be much more thorough. The reviewers may even agree to accept your work if you make certain changes or complete certain experiments. At this point you can argue with the reviewer's suggestions or simply do what they tell you to and resubmit the paper. Once the reviewers are happy with your work, the journal agrees to accept your publication and your paper may be listed on your resume as "in press."

Step 4, Page Costs

Early scientists would submit their work to organizations such as the National Academy of Science where prestigious members reviewed their work. The accepted work would then be printed and disseminated for sale. As science diverged into specialized fields it became much easier to disseminate the findings in journals which interested scientists could subscribe. This system kept researchers in any one field abreast of all the most recent developments in that field.

This is where the process becomes a bit strange and diverges from how the system was originally meant to work. Once your paper is accepted, the editor assigns your page charges. Page charges originated in order to offset the costs of editing and printing the physical journals used in the past. These charges also served to force scientists to be brief and concise in the summation of their data so that each journal wasn't 400 pages each month. Today in the typical journal a publication of 4-10 pages with no color figures will cost between $2,000 and $5,000 to publish. Unsurprisingly the page charges increase with the corresponding increase in the perceived prominence of the journal. Each color image costs between $400 and $600 to include. In the context of a printed journal, charging for color figures makes sense since color ink always costs more than black ink. Today, however, most journals are not physically printed at all. Instead, the results are converted into hyperlinked HTML and printable PDF formats. Despite the fact that converting a color figures to these formats costs no more than monochrome figures, these charges are still applied. Interestingly, since you are paying to have your work published, some journals are required by law to include a disclaimer that your research results are technically an advertisement.

I heard a talk a few years ago by a now-famous microbiologist. His research was very unusual and he had never been able to secure a single dollar in federal grant money to support his work. When he finally realized that what he had found was absolutely groundbreaking, he paid the page charges to publish his work out of his own pocket. Fortunately for him, he was right. His work on how bacterial populations can live in clouds was important in how we think about disease transmission. And his discovery that these bacteria can produce proteins that can make water turn to ice at above the freezing point changed the way that we make snow at ski resorts. I'm sure he's now a tenured full professor somewhere and gets royalties from many of the places I visit in the winter, but his story illustrates a flaw in this system. As I mention in the chapter on grants, the average age that researchers make their most significant discoveries is in their mid- 30s, nearly 10 years prior to when they will receive their first research grant. Couple that with the low salaries of postdoctoral fellows and assistant professors and you have a system in which the people who are doing the best research can't possibly afford to publish it where it will reach the largest audience. Even more frightening is this scenario: What if a major advance in cancer treatment occurs in a small college lab or at a research facility in a third-world country? Will this technique ever be made public? What if the page cost makes this innovative researcher decide to simply keep his advance to himself rather than sharing it with the world?

Step 5, Dissemination of the Research

Imagine that you've finally published your first paper. It is the crowning achievement of your scientific career. Your family is incredibly proud and happy of you. Your grandmother goes to the public library and looks up the journal hoping to read about your accomplishments, but all she can find is a short abstract. In order to read the paper that her grandson wrote, she has to pay $32.00.

This is the detail that I find the most insulting. U.S. tax dollars are disseminated to government and academic research labs. These labs perform research and use some of the tax money they receive to pay to publish this research in scientific journals. In order for the U.S. taxpayers to then access the findings of the research they paid for, all they have to do is pay $32.00 per study (or something equally ludicrous) to access the work. University libraries pay a bulk fee each year to allow their students access to a certain number of journals. I don't know what these fees are, but I'm guessing they are very large. Even when I was a government researcher working on a government facility, there were journals that I could not access because even that facility could not afford to subscribe to every research journal in my field. I have no idea how small companies or researchers at private colleges perform their research without access to the newest advancements in their area of study. Without access to the dozens (if not hundreds of journals) in your research area, how would you ever know if the research you are doing has been done by someone else – how do you know that you aren't just wasting your time, and the grant money you received...

The good news is that I'm not the only person on earth who is outraged by this system. A number of Nobel Laureates have championed the idea that all peer reviewed scientific work should become free access to the taxpayers who funded the work. Other groups have fought for allowing this work to be more easily accessed by developing countries. The latter group has had greater success to this point, meaning that I would currently be able to access more of my published work from an internet connection in China than from my local public library despite the fact that my work throughout my career has been funded by U.S. tax dollars and published exclusively in journals headquartered in the United States.

Reproducibility

As I mentioned in previous chapters, all academic researchers, as well as some government ones, are under tremendous pressure to publish. You won't obtain your Ph.D., finish your postdoctoral fellowship or become a professor anywhere without a long list of publications on your resume. Unfortunately, all of this pressure has a side effect;

at least half of the findings published in scientific journals today are not true.

I could pick one of a hundred anecdotes, but I'll describe one of the most well-known ones. A few years ago a group of researchers published a report in one of the very best journals about a new protein called STK33. The study reported that this protein was only expressed on cancer cells and that if you target that protein you will destroy the cancer cells. Pharmaceutical companies jumped on this protein, developing drugs that would destroy cells that had STK33. Nearly 6 months later, the biotech company Amgen reported that they could not reproduce any of the experiments in this study; that essentially, the findings were not true.

After the scientific community began to accept that we could no longer accept published findings as factual, Bayer pharmaceuticals decided to quantify the extent of the problem. In order to do so, Bayer picked nearly 100 studies performed in various labs around the world that were all published in the most prestigious scientific journals, and they attempted to reproduce their findings. One requirement of all journals is that you include a Methods section. This section should provide step-by-step instructions for other researchers to perform your experiments. The details must be precise, all the way to the manufacturers of every chemical and device you used in that study and how you used them. So we'd expect this to be a pretty easy job for professionals at Bayer. The results were mind-boggling: Bayer scientists were only able to reproduce 20% of the studies they selected. About 12% of the results were partially true, and over 60% of the studies were completely irreproducible. I would guess that the true number is a little lower than 60%, as the scientists at Bayer couldn't possibly be experts in every field of every paper they selected, but if you assumed that 10% was error by Bayer scientists, you still have half of the scientific literature in this small sampling being fabricated or exaggerated!

In order to curb the problem of data fabrication, most academic journals run your results through software that can detect whether your results were altered by common programs such as Photoshop. If your data is shown to contain such simple falsehoods you are typically banned from publishing in journals owned by that company for life.

An extreme case of data fabrication is currently in the news and is having repercussions on the national level. A world-leading expert in the field of genomics and professor at Duke University has been accused of fabricating nearly every study of his career. He first reported in the *New England Journal of Medicine* that his team could predict the development of lung cancer by using a technology called expression arrays. Later he reported that they could use these same arrays to tell what chemotherapies would work best for a patient. These results were so impressive that clinical trials began on real cancer patients. Expression arrays were performed on biopsies from these patients and their treatment was selected by the results of the array. Unfortunately, while the technology is a valid and valuable one, the professor had been changing the experimental results to match his predicted outcomes. The interpretation scheme was a complete fabrication which may have put these patients at risk when they could have been receiving treatment from more valid avenues. The level of fabrication in this man's career was so extreme that even his resume was found to contain falsehoods, such as the claim that he had been selected as a Rhodes Scholar. To date, seven of the publications from this group have been retracted and the professor has been removed from his position and stripped of any accolades he once received. Currently, several groups around the world are working on new methods and strategies to deter and detect fabrications of this kind. While obviously necessary, these new requirements will make it significantly more difficult for everyone performing and publishing research of this kind.

Review and Methods Books

Another place to publish data and ideas are in review and method books. These books are produced by a few mainstream publishers and come out every few months. The market is almost unparalleled on earth. Every major university and government library on earth buys every one of these books. They are commonly edited by a leader in the field being reviewed. The editor generally writes the introductory section as well as identifies suitable authors for each chapter he/she would like filled in the book. In order to be selected as an editor, you must be a clear leader in your field. Being selected or accepted as an editor for a work is a genuine honor and a great way to cement your legacy. The authors of each chapter are often postdoctoral fellows and assistant professors who are thrilled to have attracted the attention of such a prestigious editor and go to great lengths to do a good job summarizing ideas or methods used in their research.

I'll reiterate how this works: Government funded researchers contribute chapters for a book that is written in their field of study. The chapters are written by the best experts in the field using this particular technique or technology. The authors do this work in order to have evidence that they are up-and-comers in their field. The chapters are edited by a government funded leader in the field who selected the best possible authors and most important ideas and makes sure the text is coherent and of the highest quality. In return for their work, the editor receives affirmation that they are a leader in this field of study. The publisher then sells the book to government funded libraries at the reasonable price of $150-$300 per copy. See the problem? Just like the journal articles, we paid for it twice. We paid the authors to write it, and then we paid the publishers for the work. And who gets rich? The publisher who just made a couple hundred bucks a copy.

Chapter 6: The Work Force

I mentioned previously that one requirement to solving major problems in science is having the best possible work force to choose from. While there are plenty of brilliant people in science and many that are working on major diseases such as cancer, I don't think that the best people really go into medical research, and I think the chart below illustrates why that might be.

Career	Average salary	Degree	Age
Research careers			
Professor	$65k	Ph.D.	35
Postdoc	$40k	Ph.D.	28
Graduate assistant	$20k	B.S.	23
Research scientist (Ph.D.)	$75k	Ph.D.	32
Research Lab technician	$28k	B.S.	24
Research M.D.	$130k	M.D.,Ph.D.	38
Engineer (Ph.D.)	$70k	Ph.D.	30
Non Research Careers			
Medical lab technician	$45k	A.S.or B.S.	21
Engineer (B.S.)	$80k	B.S.	22
Radiology tech	$60k	A.S.or B.S.	21
Private practice M.D.	$250k	M.D.	30

Source: Summarized from multiple salary reporting services and several geographic areas.

Why We Haven't Cured Cancer

The chart above lists several arbitrarily chosen careers, along with a rough average of the salary, the required degree(s), and the age at which you could begin this career. These numbers are all rough estimates, simply listed to illustrate my point.

If you have the intelligence and the drive to truly do anything with your life, why would you subject yourself to the tortures of the biomedical sciences? As I described in the second chapter, you have few choices once beginning the path. With a bachelor's degree in biology you can go into research where you'll only be stuck doing the most menial and repetitive jobs for less than $30,000/year. If you took that same degree to a medical lab, doing the same repetitive tasks, you'd make 50% more. If you really wanted to stay in research you'd be force to endure the trials of graduate school, and probably accrue more student loan debt for your master's degree. And if you were in it for the long haul, with 4-6 years of graduate school at $20,000 a year (if you're lucky) and 2-5 years of postdoctoral work. At 32, if you were very fortunate you could finally find a job making almost as much as your classmates who completed bachelor's degrees in engineering were making 10 years previously. The most striking point to me is that a graduate with a B.S. degree in engineering typically makes more than one with a Ph.D. in the same field.

Does this sound like a system that rewards the smartest, most motivated and inventive? It doesn't to me and I certainly wouldn't recommend the career path I took to anyone that I care about, especially if they really seemed like the bright young scientists that our field so desperately needs. Fortunately, I don't need to tell these people. Every year fewer American high school students major in the biomedical sciences and fewer graduates of these programs go on to continue graduate studies in these areas.

So, where are all the scientists in the U.S. coming from? Take a look in any medical research lab in the U.S. and you'll know immediately. Like most other things in this country today, we must import our scientists from Asia, with the majority coming from China and India. Smaller numbers of researchers come from Japan, Singapore, Korea, and the Philippines. Students from these countries are often used to the grueling schedules and the amount of work that is required to complete degrees and postdoctoral fellowships in this country. And if you ask why they chose to become scientists in the U.S. you primarily get one of two slightly different answers. The first is often that they couldn't get into medical school in their home country. The second is that there are many opportunities for scientists here, while there are much fewer in their native lands.

The system in the U.S. for medical researchers is so grueling and unrewarding that no students in this country want to pursue it, so we commonly fill these openings with foreign nationals who couldn't get into the more competitive programs in their own countries. During my first postdoc I was the only native born American citizen in my lab, also the only one on the third floor, and one of three in my department of around 90 scientists (I was the only one under the age of 50, however). Don't get me wrong. Some of the best scientists (and some of the best people) I've ever known have been foreign nationals that came to the U.S. to study or to work in biomedical labs. I am not trying to demean anyone or their accomplishments. As I said previously, I doubt that I would have succeeded in the same situation. It was hard to get where I am as a U.S. citizen even with the advantages that we have here. I am asking you to question the validity of a system that requires the best and brightest, but doesn't go to lengths to recruit those within its own population.

Chapter 7: Why We Haven't Cured Cancer

Cancer is an absolutely daunting disease of incredible complexity. From nearly a century of focused research we have come up with a number of solutions and improved the outlook of patients diagnosed with a few specific cancers that affect a few specific organs. In the vast majority of cases, however, the prognosis for a cancer diagnosis isn't much better now than it was 50 years ago. Obviously we aren't looking in the right places or doing the right kinds of research. The cure for cancer is going to come from a completely different form of research or study than what we have in place currently.

Unfortunately, the system is entrenched. Instead of channeling research dollars toward new fields of study and promising new scientists with original new ideas, we waste this money. Every dollar allotted by our country to do research seems to go where it does the least amount of good. Grants are given primarily to older, established researchers whose best years of science and innovation are often well behind them. Motivated researchers with new ideas are hamstrung by the fact that the college or university that employs them takes over half of their grant money and diverts it to other uses.

Why We Haven't Cured Cancer

The cure will never come from the government research labs due to the inherent politics in these organizations and the fact that the leaders of these facilities suppress original thought and make the less senior researchers explore the field with the outdated techniques, methods, and ideas that they learned in medical school 30-40 years ago. The work that is produced by the government labs is withheld from the very public that paid for it by the long approval process from senior management officials who are both unqualified to review the work and who are more concerned with politics than in disseminating these research findings.

The cure will never come from the private sector either. The prohibitive costs of testing the cure on human patients and clinical trials discourage the research. New agents showing the highest possible potential are unlikely to be profitable enough to encourage their development when established and expensive long-term chemotherapies are still in existence.

Even if these researchers were doing the best research and were led by organizations that truly cared about curing cancer, rather than their current motivations of profit and power, another hurdle would still remain. The majority of money allotted for their research would still be diverted to corrupt scientific equipment and supply companies. If these companies are allowed to maintain their unchecked monopolies over the scientific community, eventually only a few labs will be able to afford to perform research at all. Couple this with the rapidly escalating charges to both publish and obtain scientific literature and there isn't any money left to actually pay researchers to look for the cure.

In summary, I still hope that cancer will one day be cured. I didn't write this book because I thought that this dream was impossible. I wrote this book because the system is terribly broken and only by bringing attention to the many problems will we be able to make strides toward repairing it.

In short, we need a revolution. Decades of the same old research, where we make slight improvements over the research of the past, is obviously ineffectual. If the current system was working, wouldn't we see the results by now? We need new ideas, new schools of thought, and a completely new system. We can't allow the top people in this new system to be picked simply because they were willing to accept more punishment from their superiors. And we definitely can't allow the system to be run by businessmen and politicians who have no real intentions of finding a cure and are motivated only by profits and enhancing their own status.

Why We Haven't Cured Cancer

I dream of a system where there is sufficient incentive to attract the very best students to becoming scientific researchers. This system supports the new ideas that they bring to the table and rewards them with more research dollars and tools for making progress toward new treatments for this disease. In this dream the researchers are allowed to disseminate their results to other researchers freely and move the field of cancer research in new and amazing directions. Until my dream is realized, however, I strongly believe that we will never cure cancer.

About the Author

Carl S. Bucky received his Ph.D. from a major university that you've probably heard of. He performed his postdoctoral work at two institutions that you've definitely heard of. Through the course of his career he has worked in eight separate labs and is the author of numerous original scientific works, reviews, and books. If the problems described in this book aren't resolved one day, he may one day rewrite this book with a lot more specifics (and using his real name) if he can find a loophole in the extensive non-disclosure agreements he has signed throughout his career.

www.ingramcontent.com/pod-product-compliance
Lightning Source LLC
Chambersburg PA
CBHW030905180526
45163CB00004B/1708